MW01469588

Mommy has cancer and that's okay.

Written by Virginia Whitsitt Steele

Illustrated by Chantel Barber

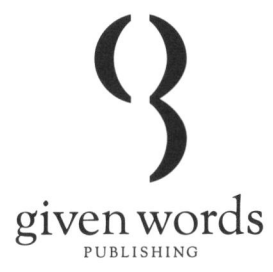

given words
PUBLISHING

Book Design & Layout: Disciple Design, Memphis, TN ©2016 Virginia Whitsitt Steele. All rights reserved.

ISBN 978-0-9973959-0-7

PRAISE FOR
"MOMMY HAS CANCER AND THAT'S OKAY."

"Telling my young children I had cancer was one of the most difficult conversations of my life. They were confused, emotional, and asked many questions I struggled to answer. "Dad, what is cancer?" "Are you going to die?" "Can the doctor make you better?" This book would have been an invaluable resource to explain complex concepts and begin the conversation which would need to occur repeatedly over the coming months. I highly recommend it for any young family coping with a recent cancer diagnosis."

Chris West
CancerKindness.com, Founder

"No author can understand fully the tears and concerns of children whose parents face cancer unless they have walked that road. Virginia Steele has been there. She has looked into her children's eyes, dried their tears and answered their questions. Now she has laid that experience out clearly and beautifully for other children. This is a book of clarity and hope that opens the way for parents to explore and address their children's fears while snuggling with a good book."

Al Weir, MD
Medical Oncologist and Hematologist, The West Cancer Center
author of When Your Doctor Has Bad News

"How I wish I had had this book during my fifty years of ministry. But not for my sake alone… for all of the children who hear those mysterious, frightening words, **Mommy has cancer***; and the adults who relate to those children. In the rhyming style of story telling a child likes, and with sensitivity and clarity, the ominous fact of cancer is presented. Add to that the fantastic art, and the child's attention is guaranteed. The definition on each page enables the adult to stay focused with a few words in answering questions children might ask. Thank you, Virginia and Chantel, children and adults are going to receive this book as a wonderful gift."*

Maxie Dunnam
Director of Christ Church Global
Senior Minister, Emeritus
Christ United Methodist Church, Memphis, TN

This book is dedicated in loving memory of my mother, Mildred Whitsitt, who showed me how to live and die with cancer.

It is also dedicated to my children, who gave me the most precious reason to conquer cancer; to celebrate their lives with them.

It is also dedicated to my loving and strong husband, Reg, who has provided me with support of all kinds and unwaveringly stands beside me empowering me to fight this fight.

And finally, it is dedicated to our precious Lord, who gives us the greatest gift of all, eternal life together.

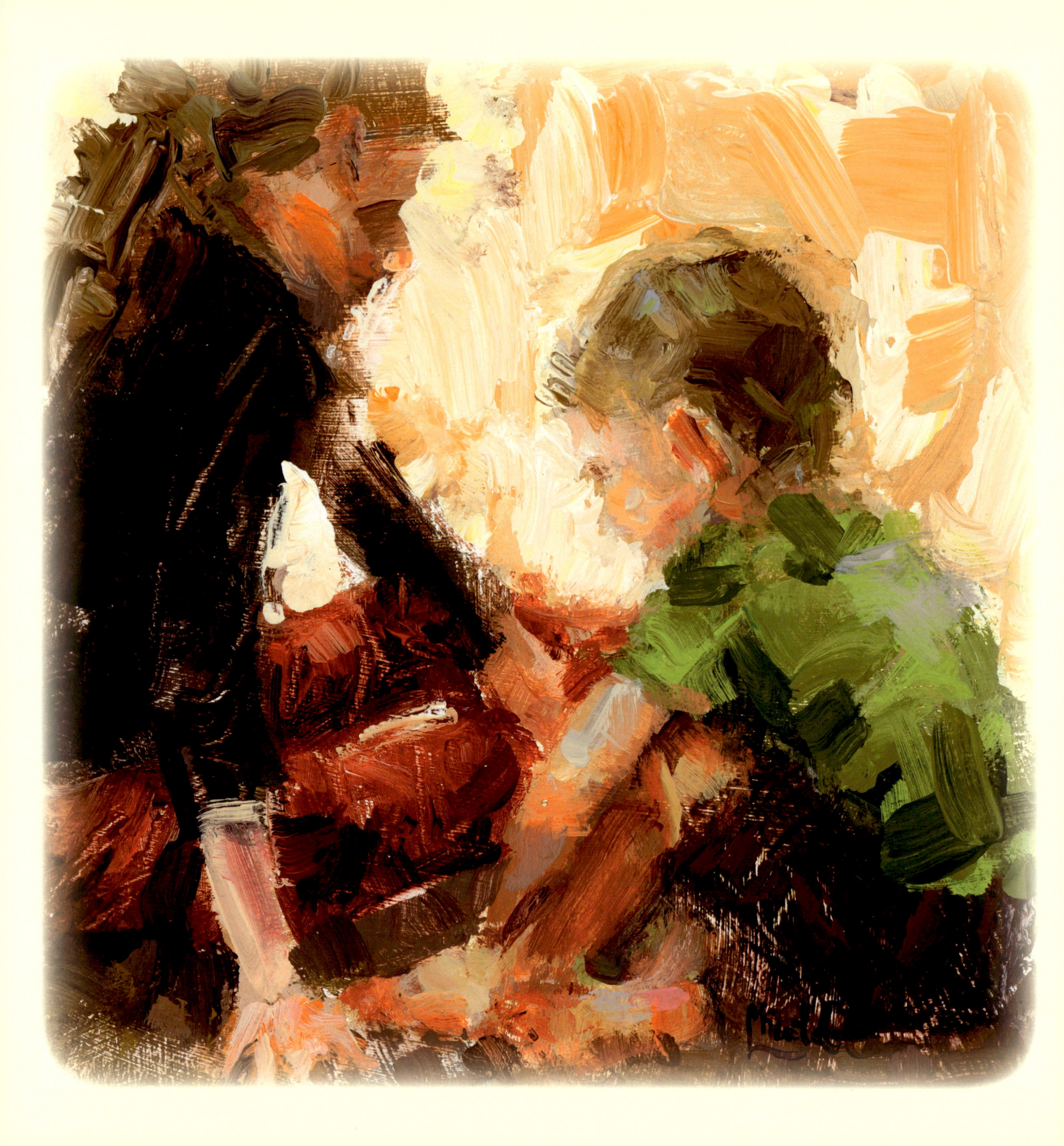

Mommy has CANCER

and that's okay,

cause she's at home with me today!

Mommy got sick and went to the

DOCTOR to see what was wrong.

He said she had cancer and told her not to wait long.

To do what he said, "Just follow our plan,

you can live with this illness,

OH YES YOU CAN!"

CANCER is when bad cells don't stop growing and hurt good cells.

A DOCTOR is a person who goes to school to learn about our body and whose job it is to take care of our health.

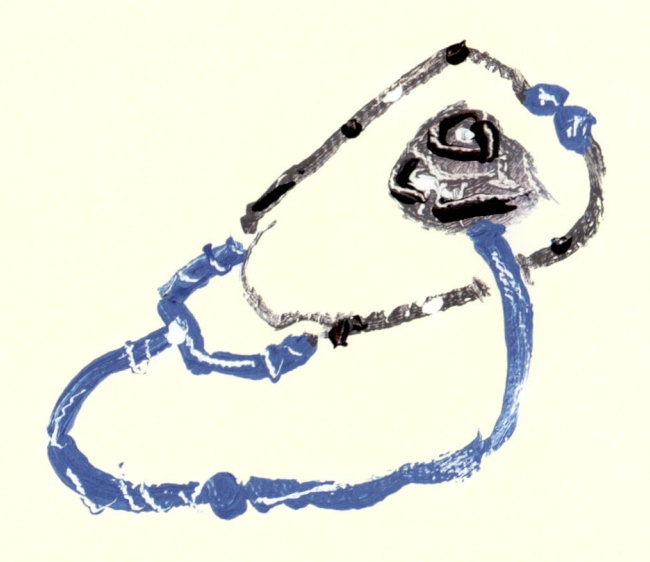

She went to the HOSPITAL, it made me sad,

I cried when she left and so did my Dad.

My little sister ran away and hid under the bed,

she covered her eyes and just shook her head.

Mommy needed an OPERATION; now what does that mean?

Daddy said it was the way a doctor makes you clean.

I asked, "Why not a bath or maybe a shower?"

But Daddy said, "NO… she needs deeper cleaning power."

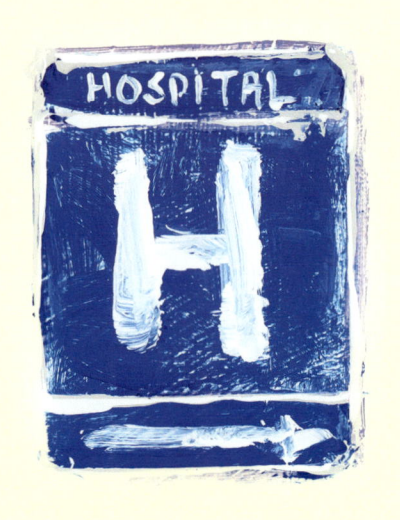

HOSPITAL is a place where doctors work and take care of patients.

OPERATION is when a doctor goes inside of your body to treat us where we are sick.

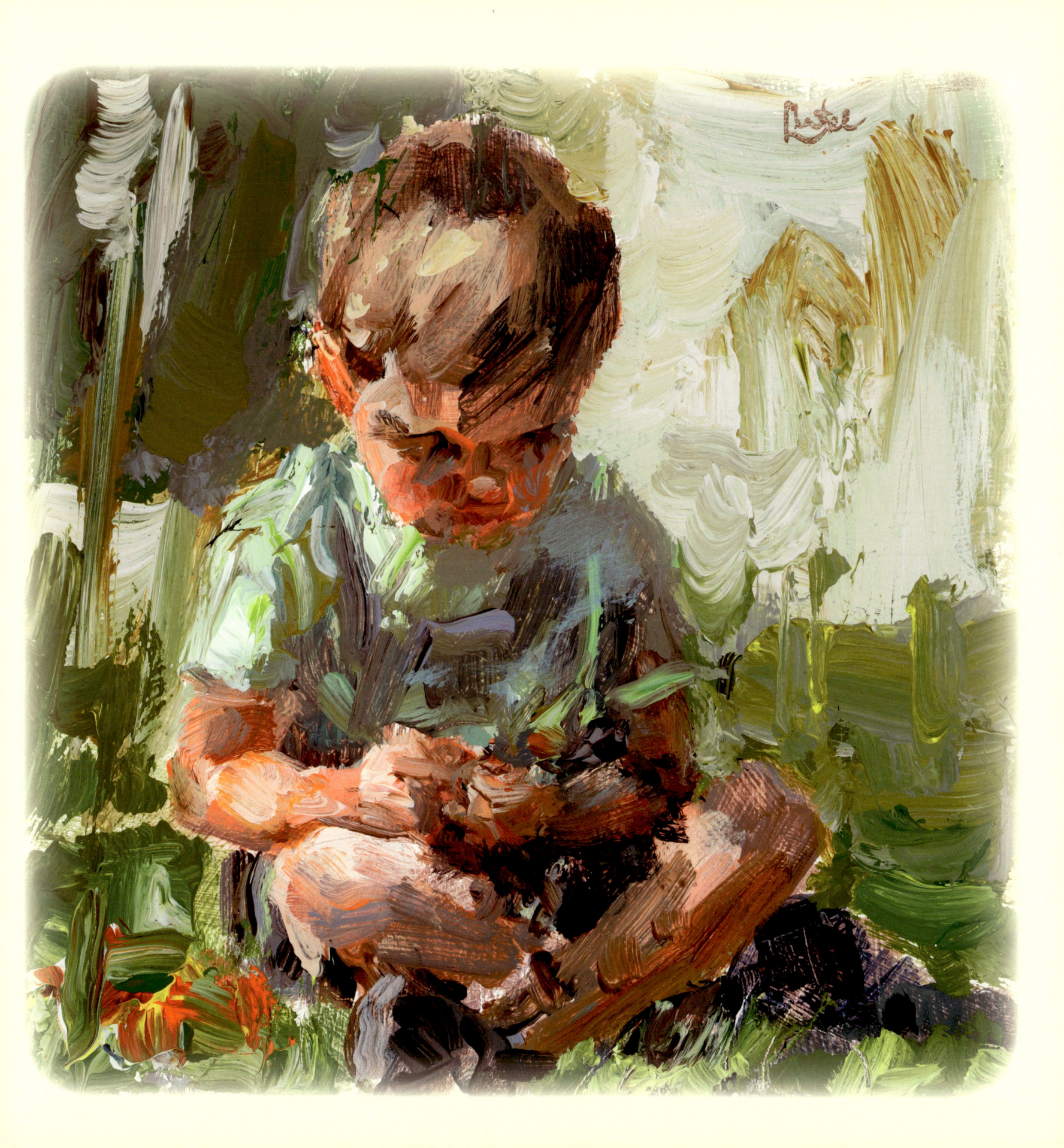

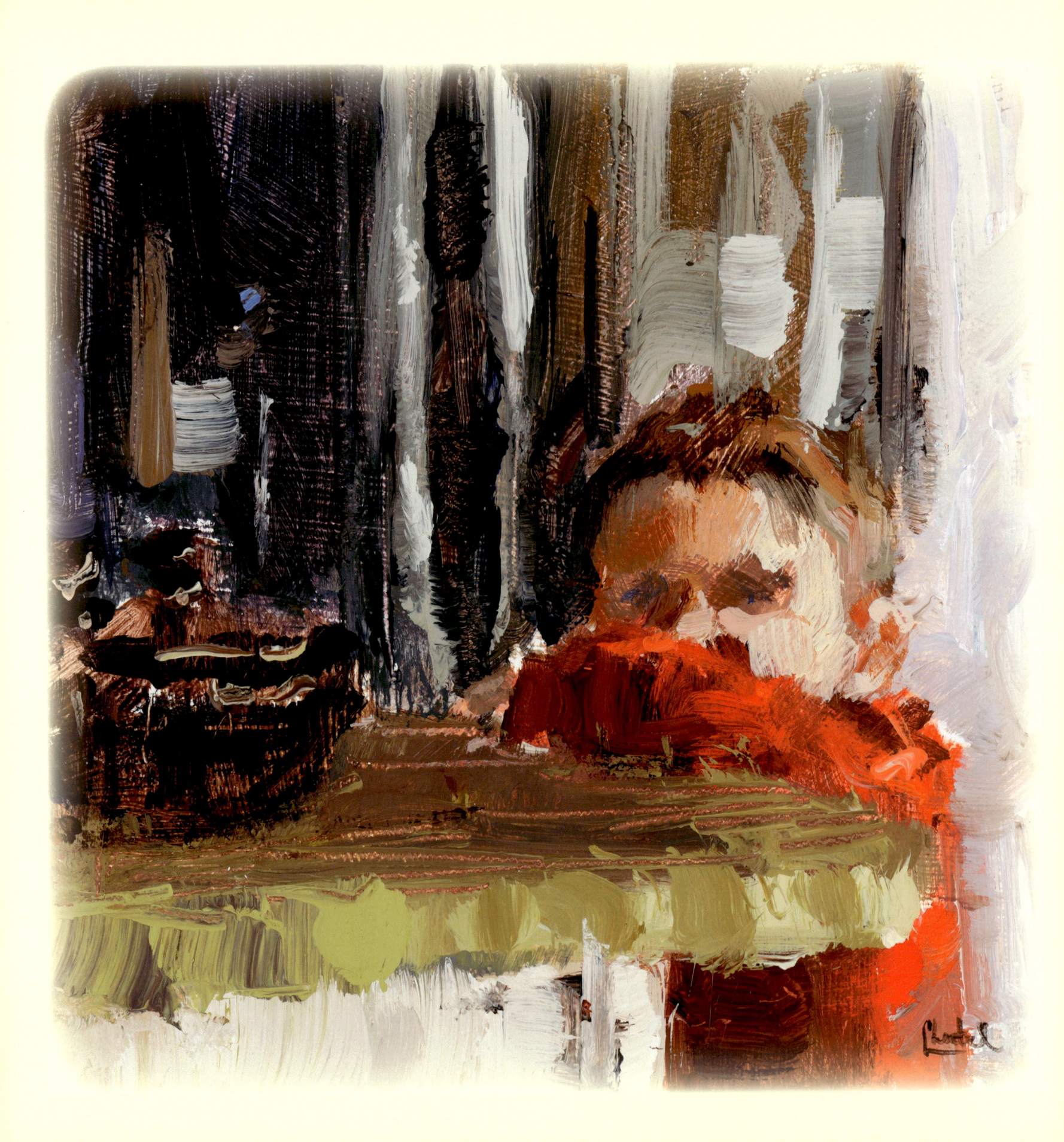

Then Grandmother and Granddaddy came to our house to stay,
Daddy went with Mommy, why did they both go away?
I just did not get it, the phone rang a lot,
people seemed sad and brought food in pots.

They talked to Grandmother and whispered all the time;
then always left saying "I know everything will be fine."
Now why did they say that? This was not fine with me,
nothing was the same as it used to be.

When Mommy was here she smiled in the morning.
While she cooked our breakfast she would always sing.
Daddy went to work and I went to school,
then she picked me up and everything was cool.

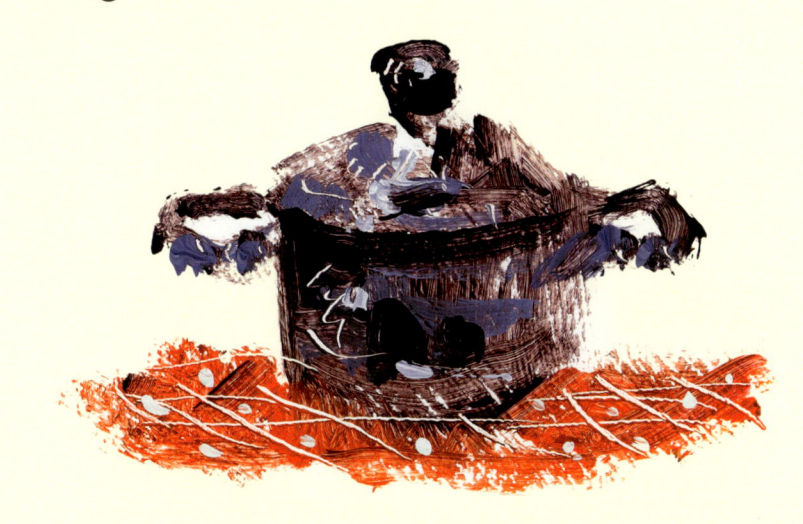

You must accept the kingdom of God as a little
child accepts things, or you will never enter it.
— Mark 10:15

Sometimes we ran errands and sometimes we napped,
then we played in the yard or I would read in her lap.
Daddy would come home and while Mommy cooked dinner
we would play ball; he called me "his little winner".

Now Mommy was gone and those people said it was fine,
well maybe at their house, but it was sure not at mine!
Finally one day Grandmother said, "Mommy is coming home."
Hooray! I was so happy I wouldn't be so alone.

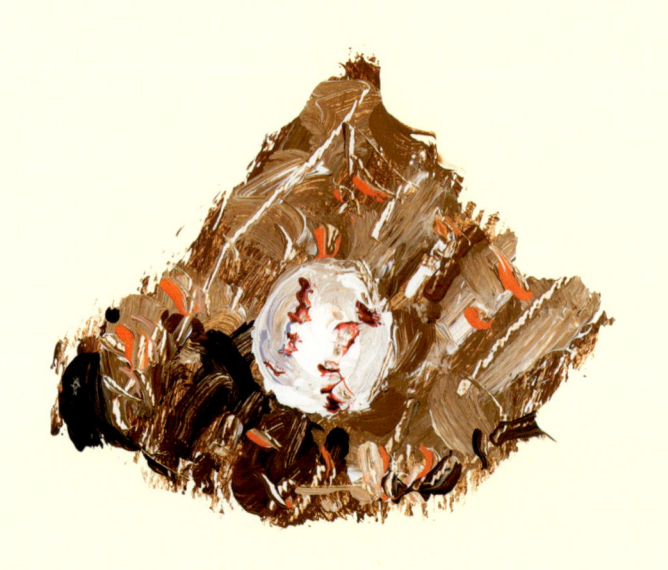

Be of good courage, and he shall strengthen
your heart, all ye that hope in the LORD.
— Psalm 31:84

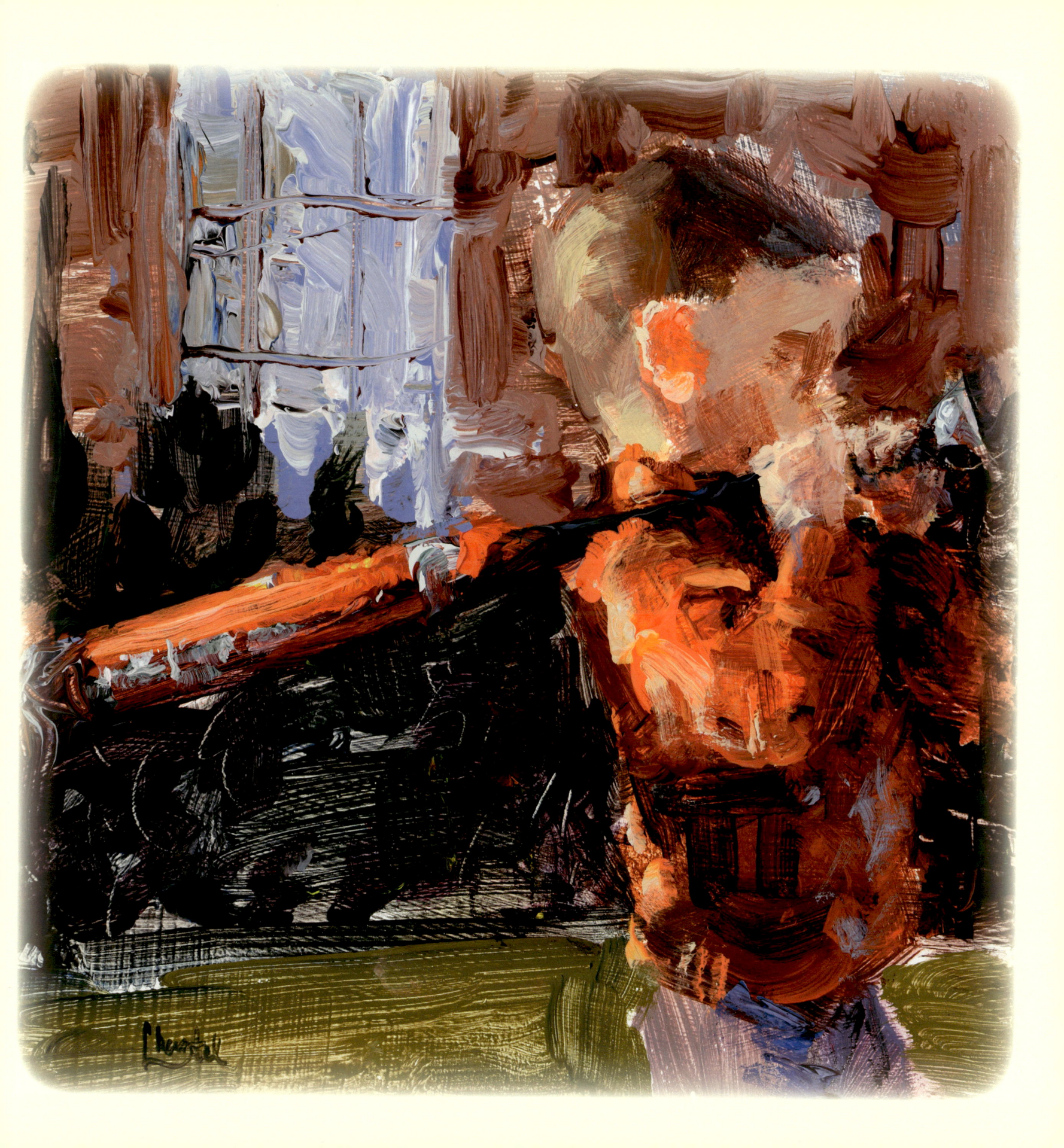

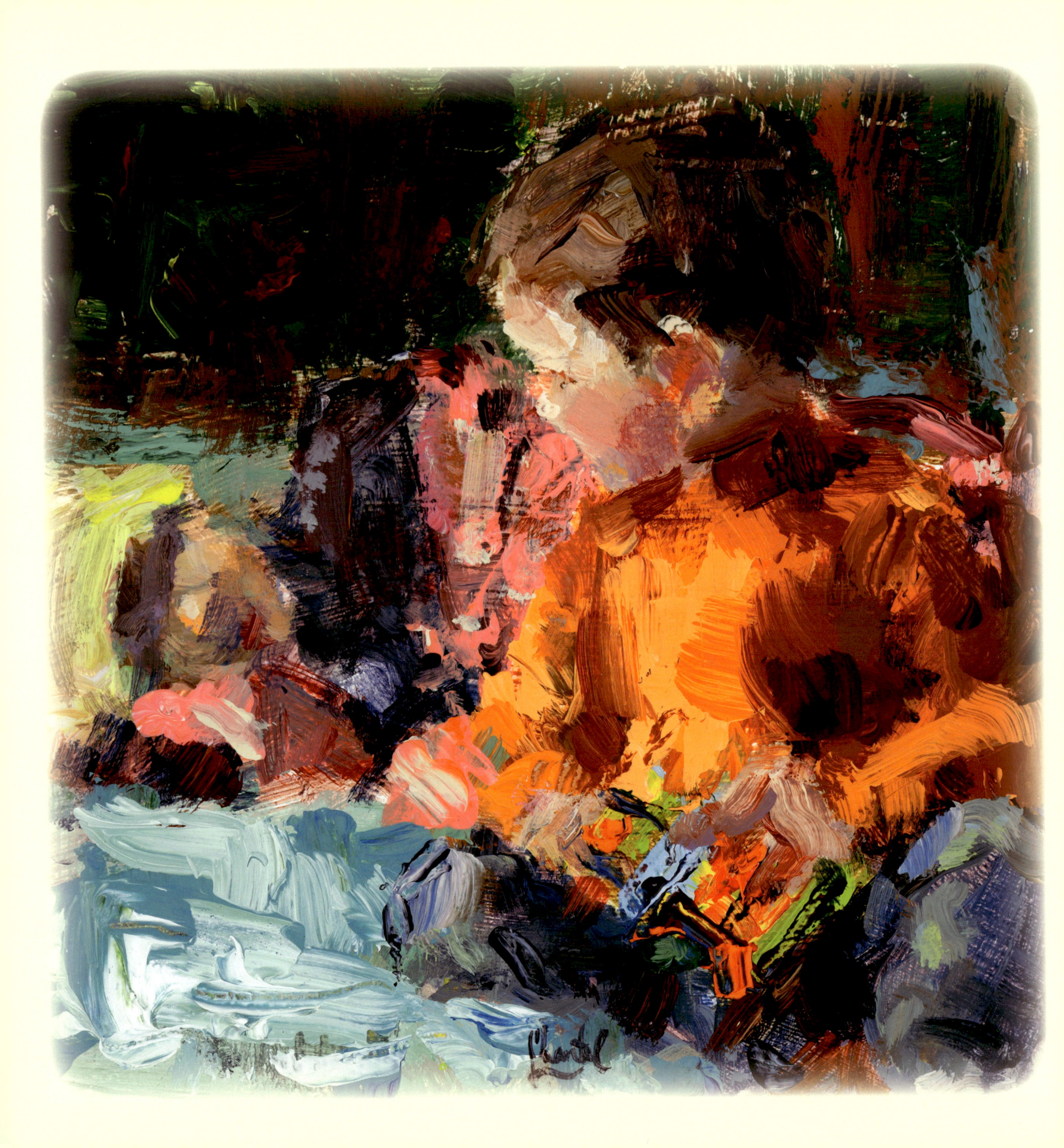

She did come home and everything was better,

now she needed to nap and I always let her.

She had to take **CHEMO**, a **MEDICINE** that made her sick.

She was pale, her hair fell out and her head was so slick.

I didn't understand why this plan was a fix;

when she left she seemed fine, but they said she was sick.

Now she seems sick and was supposed to get well?

Everyone said, "Have **FAITH** and soon you can tell."

FAITH is believing in something you cannot see or fully understand.

CHEMO is a strong medicine that can kill bad cells and sometimes the good cells too.

MEDICINE is a plant, fruit or chemical used to help us get well when we are sick.

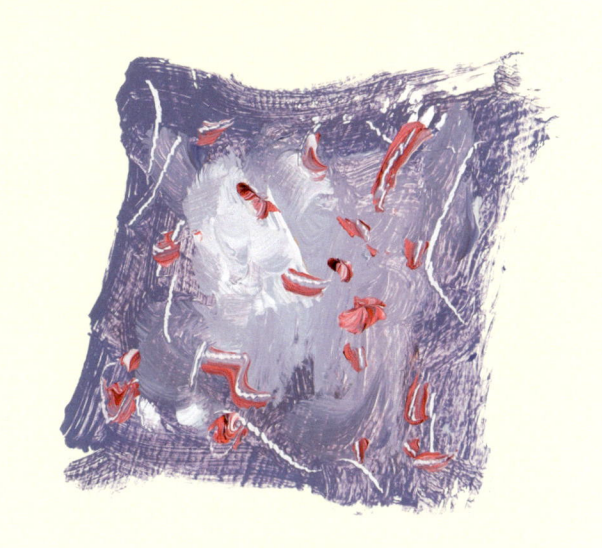

They were right and with just one more TREATMENT,
invitations to celebrate soon would be sent.
We were through with it all and I know what that means;
the plan had worked and NOW MOMMY WAS CLEAN!

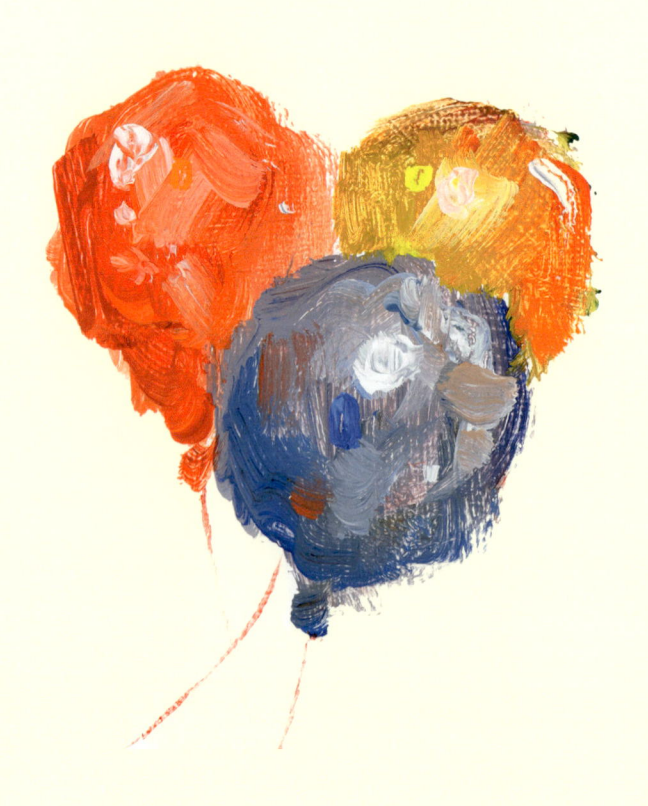

TREATMENT is a plan to take
care of any sickness.

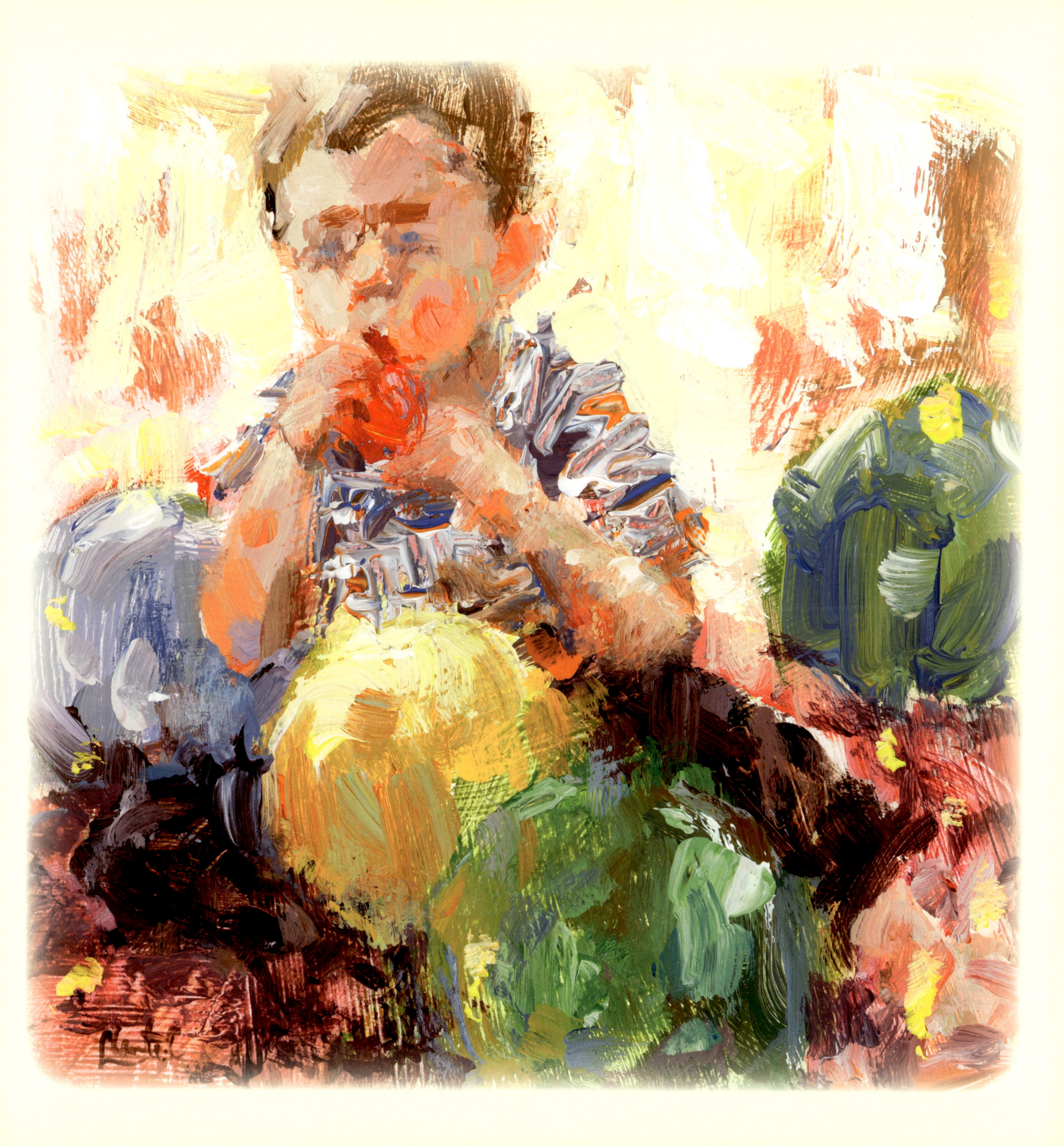

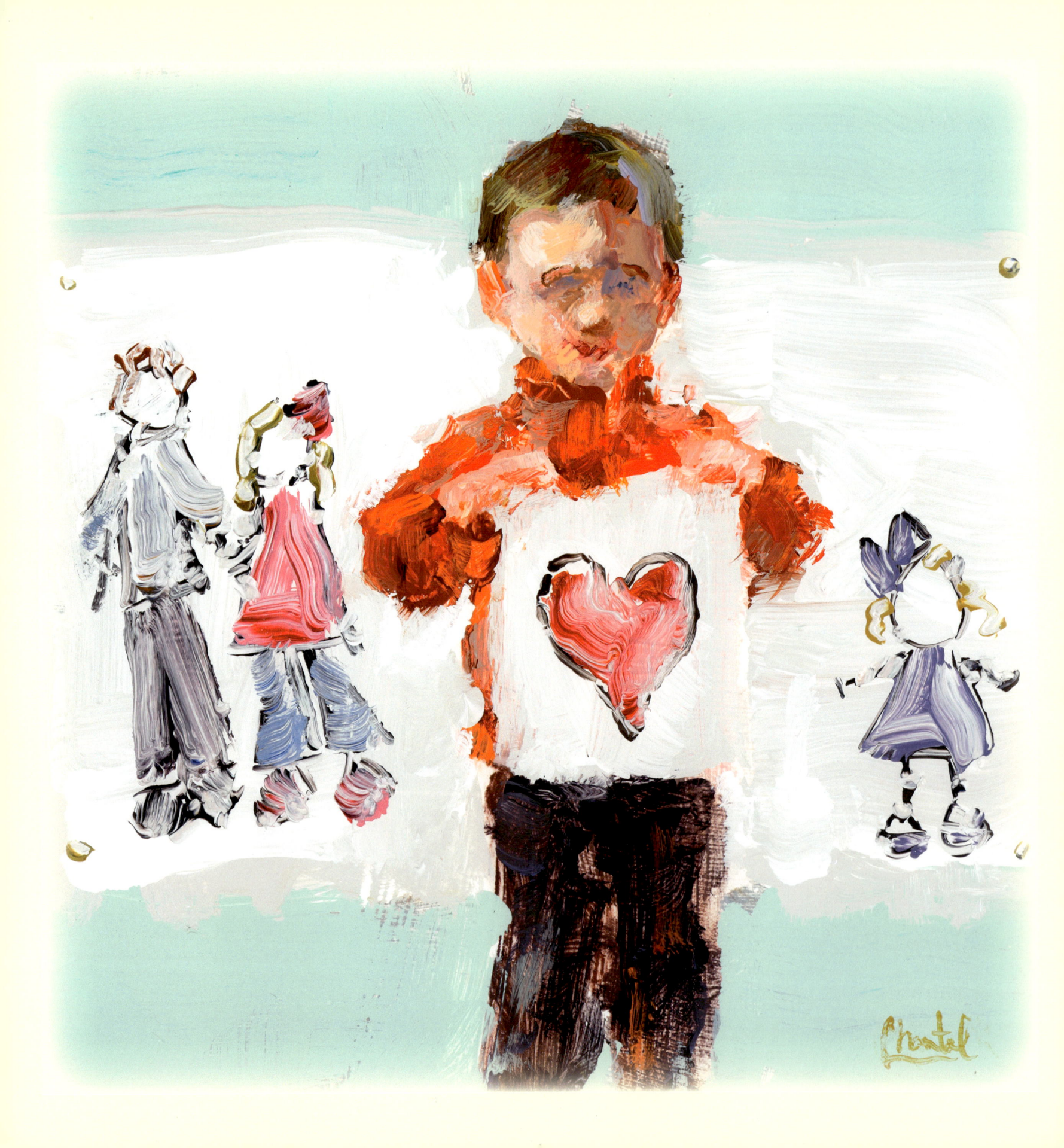

Soon Mommy felt better, my grandparents went away,

just Mommy, Sis and me, what a happy day!

Things are much better than they used to be!

We are always so happy, Mommy, Daddy, Sis and me.

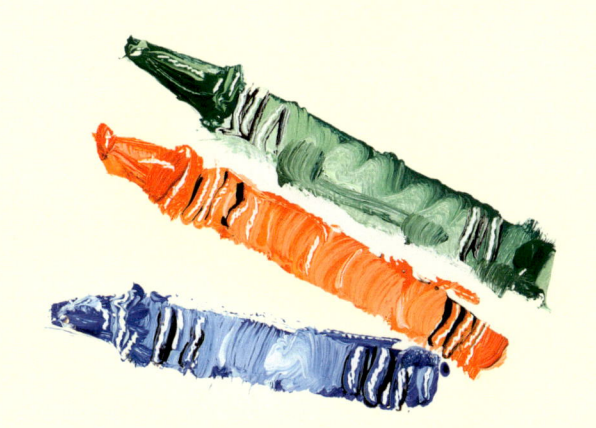

Crying may last for a night.
But joy comes in the morning.
— Psalm 30:5

We learned we have **BLESSINGS**,
those are good things from God.
Now we give thanks to our Father above;
for our home, for food, for our health, family and friends,
for each day 'til **ETERNITY**, which means
FOREVER UNTIL THE END!

**Mommy HAD cancer and that's okay,
'cause she's at home with me today.**

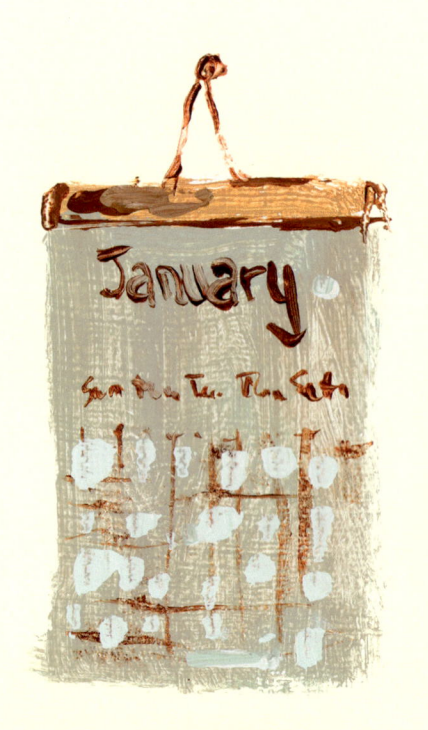

BLESSINGS are the good things we
have or that happen in our life.

ETERNITY is forever and forever,
with no end.

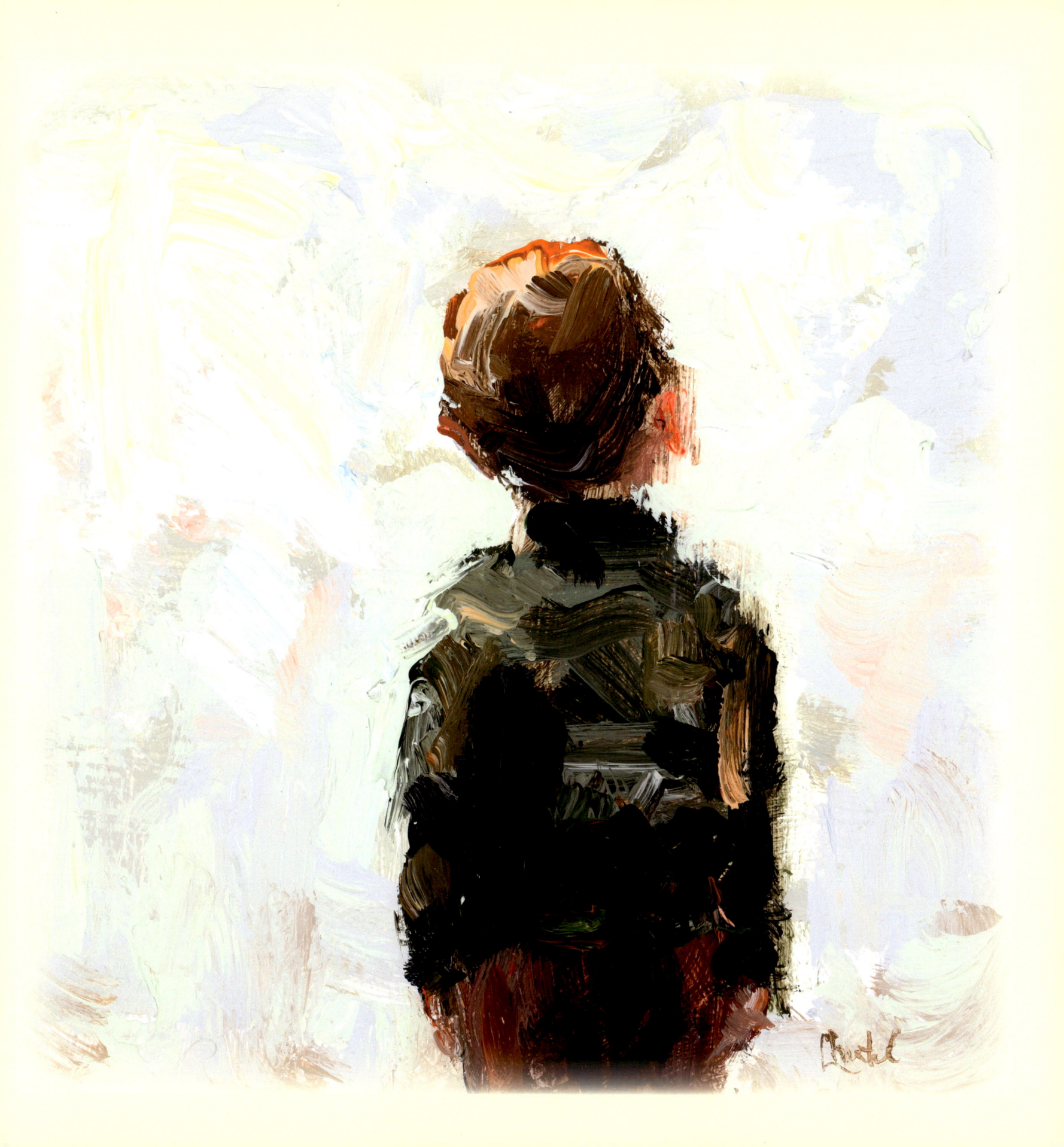

Parent's Teaching Glossary

(in order of appearance in text)

CANCER — Bad cells that don't stop growing and hurt good cells.

CELLS — The little tiny invisible pieces of our body that make up our whole body, just like sand to a beach.

DOCTOR — A person who goes to school to learn about our body and whose job it is to take care of our health.

CHECKUP — When the doctor checks our whole body for any sickness.

HOSPITAL — A place where doctors work and take care of patients.

PATIENT — A person (sick or not sick) who is being taken care of by a doctor.

SICKNESS — When your body feels bad or when it is not doing what it should do.

OPERATION   When a doctor goes inside of your body to treat us where we are sick.

CHEMO   A strong medicine that can kill bad cells and sometimes the good cells too.

MEDICINE   A plant, fruit or chemical used to help us get well when we are sick.

FAITH   Believing in something you cannot see or fully understand.

TREATMENT   A plan to take care of any sickness.

BLESSINGS   The good things we have or that happen in our life.

ETERNITY   Forever and forever, with no end.

PRAY   A way to talk to God.

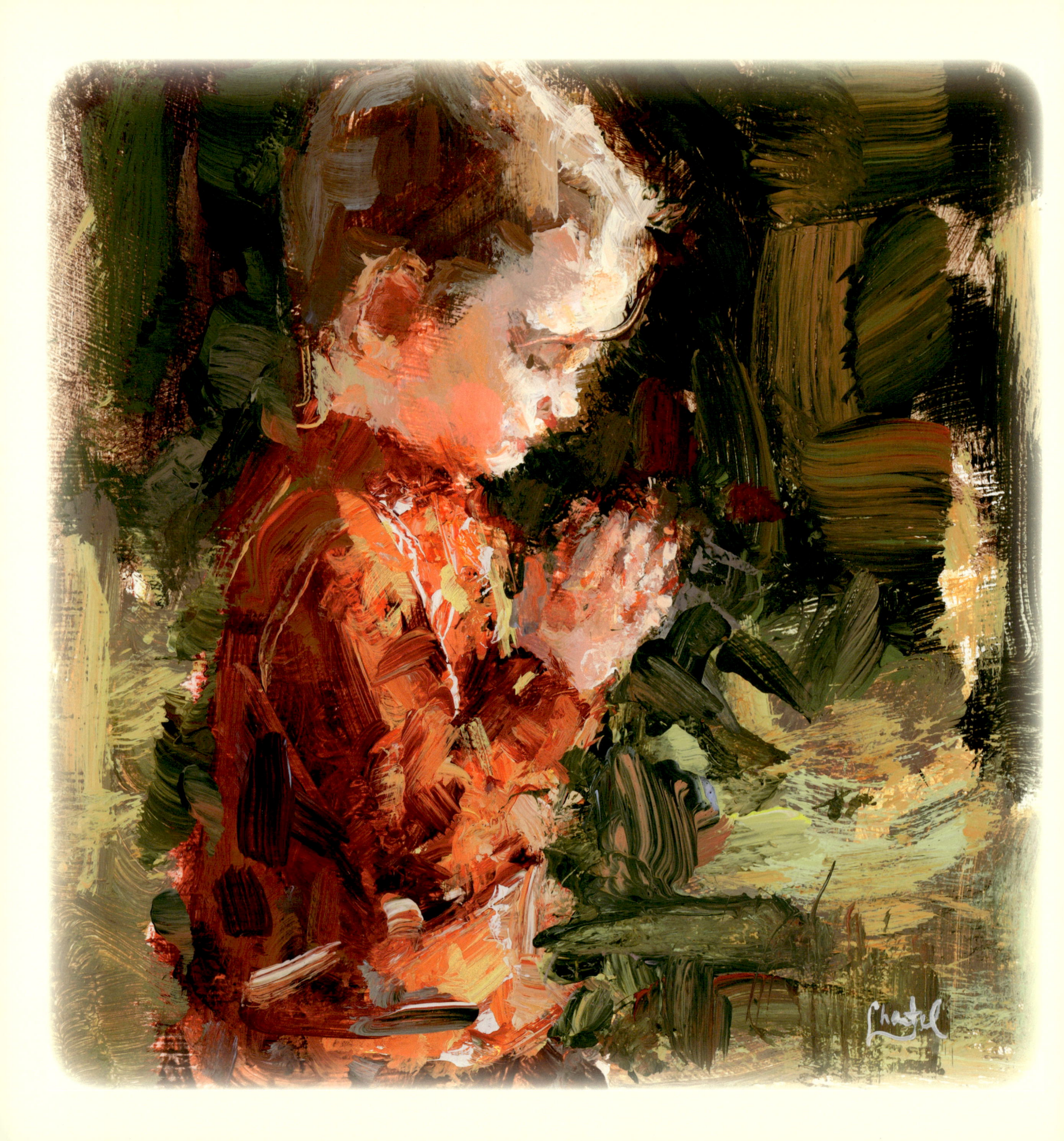

Prayer of Praise

Thank you God,

For your **LOVE**,
which gives us our family on earth.

For your **STRENGTH**,
to help us when times are hard.

For your **GIFTS**,
which gives us people who are able to help us.

For your **PEACE**,
which calms us when we are scared.

For your **WISDOM**,
so we can learn to understand.

For your **SON**,
who takes away our mistakes,

For **ETERNITY**
to always be together, forever and forever.

AMEN.

A NOTE FROM THE AUTHOR

Explaining the challenges of a cancer diagnosis, treatment and recovery, to children can be an incredibly difficult proposition. There is however good news, in that more and more often we get to tell the victory story of conquering cancer! The journey is quite challenging but the rewards are so great.

For a child this is a very overwhelming and frightening process to understand. I wrote this book when I was given a devastating cancer diagnosis and while I had very young children. I was in hope of reassuring my young son, who was so silent and so brave; whom I knew in my heart was terrified, but also curious.

I intended for this book to be read by a significant loved one, either the parent diagnosed or the parents together, the grandparents, family members or a dear friend. A message like this cannot be received by a child properly, unless it is given with love and the child is aware of being surrounded by love. With patience, time and love they will come to terms with this and grow in maturity, wisdom, compassion and kindness.

Note the opportunities for you to share these important life skills with your children:

- Honesty with others and open communication.
- Confidence and trust from ALWAYS being told the truth.
- Optimism in the face of adversity.
- Spirituality and the comfort it provides.
- God's goodness and power.
- Surrender of that which we cannot control.
- Facing fears and expressing them.
- Sibling support and love for one another.
- Friendship and its role in daily activities.
- Physicians' and good healthcare's important role in healing.
- Avoidance/denial of problems and seeking care quickly.
- Developing intellectual curiosity about new things and words.
- The power of prayer.
- The beautiful expression and feeling of joy in spite of situational unhappiness.
- Appreciation for the daily routine of our lives.
- The precious gift of each day.

Are these not life skills that many adults find lacking? Don't even mature individuals have to work on these issues daily? What a wonderful opportunity to give to a child such a firm foundation in life.

As hard as it is to believe, on the underside of cancer there are truly many blessings. I hope you will find these lessons and more in this simple story and share them with your children. They will be blessed and SO WILL YOU!